Heart conditions and treatments

Understanding Cardiovascular Health

Anita Collins

Contents

DISCLAIMER

This book is as accurate and complete as possible. There may be typographical errors or mistakes in the content. This book also contains information that is only current as of the publication date. This Book is not the definitive source of information and should only be used as a guide. The book's sole purpose is to teach. The publisher or author does not guarantee the eBook's accuracy. They are not responsible for any error, omissions, or misinformation

Introduction

The human heart is a wonderful organ that beats nonstop throughout our whole lives. Its role as the essential engine that keeps us alive allows us to continue existing. However, despite its complexity, this pump is not immune to the intricacies of human health, and disorders affecting the heart have become an increasingly prominent worry in modern society. These diseases, whether they are acquired or present at birth, can have a substantial influence on an individual's well-being and require careful attention and individualized treatment plans.

In this investigation of "Heart Conditions and Treatments," we dig into the complex terrain of cardiac health, revealing the secrets of a variety of heart-related illnesses as well as the developments in medical research that strive to restore and preserve the delicate balance of this crucial organ. Our journey spans the varied spectrum of heart diseases that affect individuals of all ages and from a variety of various backgrounds. This spectrum ranges from typical cardiovascular disorders to uncommon congenital defects.

As we progress through the many chapters of this discussion, we will not only throw light on the complexities of cardiac conditions, but we will also expose the novel therapies and therapeutic techniques that medical experts use. The arsenal against heart diseases continues to increase, bringing hope and healing to people who are currently dealing with cardiac issues. This armament includes everything from alterations to one's lifestyle and drugs to innovative surgical procedures and technology discoveries.

Overview of the Cardiovascular System

- **The heart:** A muscular pump that forces blood around the body.

- **A closed system of blood vessels:** These vessels include:

  - **Arteries:** Vessels that carry blood away from the heart.

  - **Veins:** Vessels that bring blood back to the heart.

  - **Capillaries:** Tiny vessels that branch off from arteries to deliver blood to all body tissues

There are two blood circulatory systems in the body. The first is the **systemic circulatory system**. This is the main blood circulatory system that transports blood to the organs, tissues, and cells throughout the body.

The second is the **pulmonary circulatory system**. This circulatory system moves blood between the heart and lungs. It is where oxygen enters the blood and carbon dioxide leaves the blood.

Structure of the heart

The atria and ventricles are the two top chambers of the heart, while the two lower chambers are termed the ventricles. The heart has four separate chambers. The atria and ventricles are separated by a wall, sometimes known as a "septum." The flow of blood through each of the chambers is regulated by a series of valves.

Blood follows the following through the heart:

1. Blood lacking oxygen returns from the body and enters the right atrium (upper right chamber) via the inferior vena cava and superior vena cava veins.

2. Blood flows through the tricuspid valve and enters the right ventricle (lower right chamber).

3. The right ventricle pumps blood through the pulmonary valve and out of the heart via the main pulmonary artery.

4. The blood then flows through the left and right pulmonary arteries into the lungs. Here, the process of breathing draws oxygen into the blood and removes carbon dioxide. As a result, the blood is now rich in oxygen.

5. The blood returns to the heart and flows into the left atrium (upper left chamber) via four pulmonary veins.

6. Blood flows through the mitral valve and enters the left ventricle (lower left chamber).

7. The left ventricle pumps the blood through the aortic valve into a large artery called the "aorta." This artery delivers blood to the rest of the body.

The importance of the heart

The heart pumps blood through closed vessels to every tissue within the body.

The blood itself then nutrients and oxygen to all cells in the body. Without blood, the cells and tissues would not function at their total capacity and would begin to malfunction and die.

What is the cardiac cycle?

The cardiac cycle consists of two phases.

The first phase is **diastole, in which the ventricles fill with blood**. It begins when the aortic or pulmonary valve closes and ends when the mitral or tricuspid valve closes. During diastole, blood vessels return blood to the heart in preparation for the next contraction of the ventricles.

The second phase is **systole, in which the ventricles contract and eject blood**. It begins when the mitral or tricuspid valve closes and ends when the aortic or pulmonary valve closes. The pressure inside the ventricles becomes greater than the pressure inside adjacent blood vessels, thereby forcing the blood from the ventricles to the vessels.

Common diseases of the cardiovascular system

Cardiovascular diseases can be severe and potentially life threatening. Understanding conditions that can affect the , cardiovascular system may help people seek appropriate and timely medical advice.

Overviews of some common cardiovascular diseases are below.

Heart attack

A heart attack happens when a part of the heart muscle does not receive enough blood. This can occur due to a blockage, a tear in an artery around the heart, or if the heart requires more oxygen than is available.

Symptoms of a heart attack include:

- chest pain or discomfort
- feeling lightheaded
- pain or discomfort in the jaw, neck, or back
- pain or discomfort in one or both arms or shoulders
- shortness of breath

Three of the main risk factors of a heart attack are:

- high blood cholesterol

- high blood pressure

- smoking

People who have had a heart attack can lower their chances of future cardiovascular problems by engaging in the following:

- regular physical activity

- reaching or maintaining a moderate weight

- following a heart-healthy diet

- quitting smoking

- undergoing cardiac rehabilitation

Stroke

A stroke is a medical condition in which the blood supply to a part of the brain becomes cut off. This lack of blood supply triggers the death of brain cells.

There are two types of stroke. Ischemic stroke occurs as a result of a blood clot blocking blood flow to the brain. Hemorrhagic stroke occurs as a result of a bleed in or around the brain.

Some significant risk factors of a stroke include:

- high blood pressure

- diabetes

- heart disease

- smoking

- personal or family history of stroke

- older age

- being of African American heritage

Symptoms of a stroke begin suddenly and may include:

- one-sided weakness or numbness of the leg, arm, or face

- vision problems in one or both eyes

- difficulty speaking or understanding speech

- confusion

- dizziness, loss of balance, or difficulty walking

- severe headache

The treatment for stroke will depend on the type. A person who experiences ischemic stroke may receive medications to help break up the blood clot and restore blood flow to their brain. A person who experiences a hemorrhagic stroke may require surgery to fix the blood vessel that is bleeding out.

Follow-up treatments for stroke may include:

- antiplatelet or anticoagulant medications to help prevent the formation of new blood clots

- medications to lower blood pressure

- medications called statins to reduce levels of cholesterol in the blood

- physical therapy

- rehabilitation therapy

- speech therapy

Heart failure

Heart failure occurs when the heart is unable to pump enough blood to satisfy the body's needs.

Some symptoms of heart failure include:

- persistent coughing or wheezing
- shortness of breath
- exercise intolerance
- increased heart rate
- nausea
- lack of appetite
- swelling
- fatigue
- confusion

Risk factors of heart failure include:

- high blood pressure
- coronary artery disease

- personal history of one of the following conditions:
  - heart attack
  - diabetes
  - sleep apnea
  - congenital heart defect

There is no cure for heart failure. But treatments can help to slow the progression of the disease and alleviate symptoms.

Examples include:

- lifestyle changes, such as dietary and exercise changes
- devices and surgical procedures
- medications to manage blood pressure or cholesterol levels
- diuretics to reduce swelling, or edema

Arrhythmia

An arrhythmia is an abnormal heart rhythm. It may present as a heartbeat that is too quick, too slow, or has a distinctive pattern. Symptoms may include:

- fast or slow heartbeat
- skipping beats
- lightheadedness
- dizziness
- fainting
- chest pain
- shortness of breath
- sweating

The risk factors of arrhythmia include:

- heart disease
- congenital heart defect
- high blood pressure
- high cholesterol
- older age
- alcohol use
- untreated sleep apnea

Importance of Heart Health

Because of the important function it performs in maintaining our lives, the heart is considered an essential organ. It circulates blood throughout our whole body, ensuring that all of our organs and tissues get the oxygen and nutrients they need to continue to be healthy and perform their functions correctly. Maintaining the health of the heart, which is a component of the cardiovascular and circulation system, is extremely important. This necessitates adopting preventative steps to ensure that the heart muscle is built up and stays healthy for a longer and more fulfilling life.

Eating well, being active, and having frequent checkups with your physician to ensure there are no problems and, in the event that there are problems, being able to address them right away all contribute to having a healthy heart. Participating in these activities maintains a healthy heart and lowers the risk of developing cardiac diseases that might lead to more serious issues or even emergency situations.

Diseases of the heart are the top cause of mortality for both men and women; in fact, one person passes away from a heart disease-related reason every 36 seconds. It is predicted that around $219 billion will be spent each year to manage or keep a cardiac problem under control.

It's also essential to keep in mind that a heart attack is only one symptom of heart illness. Heart disease encompasses a wide range of disorders in addition to a heart attack, including coronary artery disease (CAD), heart infections, heart failure, angina, peripheral arterial disease (PAD), and other conditions. There are benefits to taking care of your heart health over the long term, even though many of these conditions can be managed and are not considered to pose a high risk for an emergency or to be life-threatening. Not only does doing so reduce the likelihood of developing heart conditions as we get older, but it also reduces the risk of developing chronic conditions that require ongoing treatment with medications.

While we could certainly add more to this list, here are our top three benefits of having **a healthy heart:**

1. Lower blood pressure

Your blood pressure is measured as the force of the blood pressing against the arterial walls throughout your body. Your blood must travel via your arteries in order to reach your heart and all of the other components of your body. When this is affected, symptoms or disorders may reveal themselves and have an influence on your general health. This can happen whether your blood pressure is low or high. The majority of people acquire high blood pressure over a period of time, and it is often the result of leading an unhealthy lifestyle, which causes damage to your internal organs, most notably your heart. If you take care of yourself and keep an eye on your blood pressure, you can lower your chances of developing high blood pressure and heart failure.

Because your blood pressure is so significant, it is measured using two numbers: your systolic blood pressure, which is the force that your blood exerts against the artery wall when your heart beats, and your diastolic blood pressure, which is the pressure that your blood exerts against the artery wall when your heart is at rest. A normal range for systolic blood pressure is less than 120 mm Hg, while a normal range for diastolic blood pressure is less than 80 mm Hg.

2. Prevent high or low blood sugar and insulin levels

Our bodies derive their energy from glucose, most commonly referred to as sugar. Throughout the day, our ability to operate is greatly dependent on it. But symptoms start to appear, which might have a severe impact on our health if there is not enough sugar in the body or if there is too much sugar in the body. Headaches and lightheadedness are two of the most prevalent early warning symptoms of low blood sugar, which indicates that your body's supply of energy is running dangerously low.

The opposite end of the scale is hyperglycemia, which in most cases requires insulin treatment to bring it under control. On the other hand, a person's own natural insulin might be impacted, which would lead to an increase in their blood sugar levels. If they increase too rapidly, it may result in a dip in the amount of sugar in your blood.

Even while our bodies are quite good at controlling the levels of blood sugar in our bodies, there are instances when age, certain health issues, and certain lifestyle behaviors can interfere with this natural process. Maintaining a healthy balance of blood sugar can be challenging. Although we don't require an excessive amount of glucose, we also can't have too little of it. What we put in our bodies has a direct influence on how much sugar we consume and how we get it. Food is a source of nutrients, but if we aren't careful about what we eat for example, if we consume an excessive amount of sugar we can have a negative impact on our health. This can lead to chronic health conditions such as hyperglycemia, diabetes, kidney failure, heart and blood vessel disease, and an increased risk of heart attacks or strokes.

3. Reduce the risk of heart attacks

The volume of blood that our heart receives is an important factor in determining its overall health. When there is an accumulation of fat, cholesterol, or plaque in the bloodstream, the volume of blood that the heart gets is reduced. This can lead to heart failure. In some circumstances, a blood clot may develop and obstruct the flow of blood, therefore reducing the volume of blood that is delivered to the heart. When our organs and tissues do not receive the adequate blood flow, they are effectively deprived of oxygen and begin the process of dying. This occurs when our circulatory system is compromised.

Although there are drugs that can help prevent heart attacks and reduce the chance of developing heart disease, it is never too late to lessen or take preventative actions to curb situations that may lead to this potentially catastrophic emergency. You may prevent difficulties that frequently occur with aging if you take care of your heart by maintaining a nutritious diet, engaging in regular exercise, and cutting back on your consumption of cigarettes and alcohol. Even while advances in modern medicine have made significant strides toward improving cardiovascular health, if it is something that can be avoided entirely, we should make it a priority to do all in our power to ensure that we live longer, healthier lives with content hearts.

Common Heart Conditions

Coronary Artery Disease (CAD)

Coronary artery disease is one of the most frequent forms of heart disease. It is difficult for the coronary arteries, which are the primary blood vessels that supply the heart, to deliver adequate amounts of blood, oxygen, and nutrients to the heart muscle. Inflammation and the buildup of cholesterol deposits called plaques in the coronary arteries are often the root causes of coronary artery disease.

When the heart does not receive an adequate supply of oxygen-rich blood, signs and symptoms of coronary artery disease might become apparent. Chest discomfort, often known as angina, and shortness of breath can be symptoms of coronary artery disease. Both of these conditions are caused by a reduction in blood supply to the heart. A heart attack may be the result of the circulation of blood being completely obstructed.

The development of coronary artery disease frequently takes several decades. It is possible that symptoms will go unrecognized until either a large blockage creates issues or a heart attack takes place. The development of coronary artery disease can be avoided by adopting a lifestyle that is beneficial to the heart.

Symptoms

In the beginning, symptoms could not be identified, or they might only appear when the person's heart is pumping rapidly, such as while they are exercising. The coronary arteries continue to narrow, which results in a decreased amount of blood reaching the heart, which in turn can cause symptoms to become more severe or frequent.

Coronary artery disease signs and symptoms can include:

- **Chest pain (angina).** You may feel pressure or tightness in your chest. Some people say it feels like someone is standing on their chest. The chest pain usually occurs on the middle or left side of the chest. Activity or strong emotions can trigger angina. The pain usually goes away within minutes after the triggering event ends. In some people, especially women, the pain may be brief or sharp and felt in the neck, arm or back.

- **Shortness of breath.** You may feel like you can't catch your breath.

- **Fatigue.** If the heart can't pump enough blood to meet your body's needs, you may feel unusually tired.

- **Heart attack.** A completely blocked coronary artery will cause a heart attack. The classic signs and symptoms of a heart attack include crushing chest pain or pressure, shoulder or arm pain, shortness of breath, and sweating. Women may have less typical symptoms, such as neck or jaw pain, nausea and fatigue. Some heart attacks don't cause any noticeable signs or symptoms.

Causes and Risk Factors

The development of coronary artery disease is preceded by the accumulation of fatty deposits, cholesterol, and other chemicals on the inner walls of the coronary arteries. Atherosclerosis is the name given to this ailment. Plaque is the name given to the accumulation. Plaque has the potential to constrict the arteries, which would impede blood flow. It's also possible for the plaque to burst, which would result in a clot of blood forming.

Besides high cholesterol, damage to the coronary arteries may be caused by:

- Diabetes or insulin resistance

- High blood pressure

- Not getting enough exercise (sedentary lifestyle)

- Smoking or tobacco use

Diagnostic Procedures

To diagnose coronary artery disease, a health care provider will examine you. You'll likely be asked questions about your medical history and any symptoms. Blood tests are usually done to check your overall health.

Tests

Test to help diagnose or monitor coronary artery disease include:

- **Electrocardiogram (ECG or EKG).** This quick and painless test measures the electrical activity of the heart. It can show how fast or slow the heart is beating. Your provider can look at signal patterns to determine if you're having or had a heart attack.

- **Echocardiogram.** This test uses sound waves to create pictures of the beating heart. An echocardiogram can show how blood moves through the heart and heart valves.

Parts of the heart that move weakly may be caused by a lack of oxygen or a heart attack. This may be a sign of coronary artery disease or other conditions.

- **Exercise stress test.** If signs and symptoms occur most often during exercise, your provider may ask you to walk on a treadmill or ride a stationary bike during an ECG. If an echocardiogram is done while you do these exercises, the test is called a stress echo. If you can't exercise, you might be given medications that stimulate the heart like exercise does.

- **Nuclear stress test.** This test is similar to an exercise stress test but adds images to the ECG recordings. A nuclear stress test shows how blood moves to the heart muscle at rest and during stress. A radioactive tracer is given by IV. The tracer helps the heart arteries show up more clearly on images.

- **Heart (cardiac) CT scan.** A CT scan of the heart can show calcium deposits and blockages in the heart arteries.

Calcium deposits can narrow the arteries.

Sometimes dye is given by IV during this test. The dye helps create detailed pictures of the heart arteries. If dye is used, the test is called a CT coronary angiogram.

- **Cardiac catheterization and angiogram.** During cardiac catheterization, a heart doctor (cardiologist) gently inserts a flexible tube (catheter) into a blood vessel, usually in the wrist or groin. The catheter is gently guided to the heart. X-rays help guide it. Dye flows through the catheter. The dye helps blood vessels show up better on the images and outlines any blockages.

If you have an artery blockage that needs treatment, a balloon on the tip of the catheter can be inflated to open the artery. A mesh tube (stent) is typically used to keep the artery open.

Treatment Options

Changes in lifestyle, such as giving up smoking, eating better, and getting more exercise, are typically recommended as part of the treatment for coronary artery disease. There are occasions when medical treatments and drugs are required.

Medications

There are many drugs available to treat coronary artery disease, including:

- **Cholesterol drugs.** Medications can help lower bad cholesterol and reduce plaque buildup in the arteries. Such drugs include statins, niacin, fibrates and bile acid sequestrants.

- **Aspirin.** Aspirin helps thin the blood and prevent blood clots. Daily low-dose aspirin therapy may be recommended for the primary prevention of heart attack or stroke in some people.

Daily use of aspirin can have serious side effects, including bleeding in the stomach and intestines. Don't start taking a daily aspirin without talking to your health care provider.

- **Beta blockers.** These drugs slow the heart rate. They also lower blood pressure. If you've had a heart attack, beta blockers may reduce the risk of future attacks.

- **Calcium channel blockers.** One of these drugs may be recommended if you can't take beta blockers or beta blockers don't work. Calcium channel blockers can help improve symptoms of chest pain.

- **Angiotensin-converting enzyme (ACE) inhibitors and angiotensin II receptor blockers (ARBs).** These medicines lower blood pressure. They may help keep coronary artery disease from getting worse.

- **Nitroglycerin.** This medicine widens the heart arteries. It can help control or relieve chest pain. Nitroglycerin is available as a pill, spray or patch.

- **Ranolazine.** This medication may help people with chest pain (angina). It may be prescribed with or instead of a beta blocker.

Heart Failure

When the heart muscle is unable to pump blood as effectively as it should, a condition known as heart failure can develop. When anything like this takes place, the body's blood supply frequently reverses, and fluid can accumulate in the lungs, leading to a sensation of being unable to catch one's breath.

Certain cardiac disorders might progressively render the heart incapable of effectively filling and pumping blood because it becomes too weak or stiff. A narrowing of the arteries in the heart and excessive blood pressure are two examples of these disorders.

The symptoms of heart failure can sometimes be alleviated with the right medication, which can also help some patients live longer. Alterations to one's way of life can boost one's quality of life. Make an effort to get more exercise, cut back on salt intake, and reduce your overall body fat.

However, heart failure is a potentially fatal condition. People who suffer from heart failure frequently exhibit significant symptoms. A heart transplant or another device to assist the heart in its function as a pump may be necessary for some patients.

Types of Heart Failure

Heart failure often affects just one side of the heart, either the left or the right, but it can sometimes affect both sides. Accordingly, cardiologists distinguish between three distinct forms of heart failure, which are as follows:

- **Left-sided heart failure**: The left ventricle of the heart no longer pumps enough blood around the body. As a result, blood builds up in the pulmonary veins (the blood vessels that carry blood away from the lungs). This causes shortness of breath, trouble breathing or coughing – especially during physical activity. Left-sided heart failure is the most common type.

- **Right-sided heart failure:** Here the right ventricle of the heart is too weak to pump enough blood to the lungs. This causes blood to build up in the veins (the blood vessels that carry blood from the organs and tissue back to the heart). The increased pressure inside the veins can push fluid out of the veins into surrounding tissue. This leads to a build-up of fluid in the legs, or less commonly in the genital area, organs or the abdomen (belly).

- **Biventricular heart failure:** In biventricular heart failure, both sides of the heart are affected. This can cause the same symptoms as both left-sided and right-sided heart failure, such as shortness of breath and a build-up of fluid.

These days, heart failure is characterized more and more on the basis of how well the heart can pump blood throughout the body. This is due to the fact that the pumping ability plays a significant part in determining which drug is the most appropriate.

There are two different kinds of heart failure that can occur here:

- **Heart failure with reduced pumping ability**: The heart muscle has become weaker, and no longer pumps enough blood around the body when it contracts (squeezes). As a result, the organs in the body don't get enough oxygen. The medical term for this is "heart failure with reduced ejection fraction."

- **Heart failure with preserved pumping ability**: Although the heart muscle is still strong, it can no longer relax and widen enough after it has squeezed blood out, so it doesn't fill up with blood properly. Despite pumping strongly enough, not enough blood is pumped out into the body as a result, especially during physically strenuous activities. Doctors call this "heart failure with preserved ejection fraction."

Signs and Symptoms

When you have heart failure, your heart is unable to pump enough blood to satisfy the demands of the rest of your body.

The manifestation of symptoms could take its time. The signs of heart failure can sometimes appear out of nowhere. Some of the signs of heart failure include:

- Shortness of breath with activity or when lying down.

- Fatigue and weakness.

- Swelling in the legs, ankles and feet.

- Rapid or irregular heartbeat.

- Reduced ability to exercise.

- Wheezing.

- A cough that doesn't go away or a cough that brings up white or pink mucus with spots of blood.

- Swelling of the belly area.

- Very rapid weight gain from fluid buildup.

- Nausea and lack of appetite.

- Difficulty concentrating or decreased alertness.

- Chest pain if heart failure is caused by a heart attack.

Causes

Heart failure can be caused by a weakened, damaged or stiff heart.

- If the heart is damaged or weakened, the heart chambers may stretch and get bigger. The heart can't pump out the needed amount of blood.

- If the main pumping chambers of the heart, called the ventricles, are stiff, they can't fill with enough blood between beats.

The heart muscle can be damaged by certain infections, heavy alcohol use, illegal drug use and some chemotherapy medicines. Your genes also can play a role.

Any of the following conditions also can damage or weaken the heart and cause heart failure.

- **Coronary artery disease and heart attack.** Coronary artery disease is the most common cause of heart failure. The disease results from the buildup of fatty deposits in the arteries. The deposits narrow the arteries. This reduces blood flow and can lead to heart attack.

A heart attack occurs suddenly when an artery feeding the heart becomes completely blocked. Damage to the heart muscle from a heart attack may mean that the heart can no longer pump as well as it should.

- **High blood pressure.** Also called hypertension, this condition forces the heart to work harder than it should to pump blood through the body. Over time, the extra work can make the heart muscle too stiff or too weak to properly pump blood.

- **Heart valve disease.** The valves of the heart keep blood flowing the right way. If a valve isn't working properly, the heart must work harder to pump blood. This can weaken the heart over time. Treating some types of heart valve problems may reverse heart failure.

- **Inflammation of the heart muscle, also called myocarditis.** Myocarditis is most commonly caused by a virus, including the COVID-19 virus, and can lead to left-sided heart failure.

- **A heart problem that you're born with, also called a congenital heart defect.** If the heart and its chambers or valves haven't formed correctly, the other parts of the heart have to work harder to pump blood. This may lead to heart failure.

- **Irregular heart rhythms, called arrhythmias.** Irregular heart rhythms may cause the heart to beat too fast, creating extra work for the heart. A slow heartbeat also may lead to heart failure. Treating an irregular heart rhythm may reverse heart failure in some people.

- **Other diseases.** Some long-term diseases may contribute to chronic heart failure. Examples are diabetes, HIV infection, an overactive or underactive thyroid, or a buildup of iron or protein.

Causes of sudden heart failure also include:

- Allergic reactions.

- Any illness that affects the whole body.

- Blood clots in the lungs.

- Severe infections.

- Use of certain medicines.

- Viruses that attack the heart muscle.

Heart failure usually begins with the lower left heart chamber, called the left ventricle. This is the heart's main pumping chamber. But heart failure also can affect the right side. The lower right heart chamber is called the right ventricle. Sometimes heart failure affects both sides of the heart.

Prevention

Treating and keeping under control the factors that might lead to heart failure is one method for the prevention of this condition. Conditions such as coronary artery disease, high blood pressure, diabetes, and obesity are included in this category.

Some of the same lifestyle changes used to manage heart failure also may help prevent it. Try these heart-healthy tips:

- Don't smoke.

- Get plenty of exercise.

- Eat healthy foods.

- Maintain a healthy weight.

- Reduce and manage stress.

- Take medicines as directed.

Treatment Approaches

The treatment of heart failure may vary according on the underlying cause. Alterations to one's way of life and medicinal intervention are frequently components of treatment. If there is another medical issue that is causing heart failure, addressing that illness may be able to reverse heart failure.

Some patients who have heart failure require surgery in order to have clogged arteries unblocked or to implant a device that will assist the heart in working more effectively.

Improvement in symptoms of heart failure is possible with medication.

Medications

A combination of medicines may be used to treat heart failure. The specific medicines used depend on the cause of heart failure and the symptoms. Medicines to treat heart failure include:

- **Angiotensin-converting enzyme (ACE) inhibitors.** These drugs relax blood vessels to lower blood pressure, improve blood flow and decrease the strain on the heart. Examples include enalapril (Vasotec, Epaned), lisinopril (Zestril, Qbrelis) and captopril.

- **Angiotensin II receptor blockers (ARBs).** These drugs have many of the same benefits as ACE inhibitors. They may be an option for people who can't tolerate ACE inhibitors. They include losartan (Cozaar), valsartan (Diovan) and candesartan (Atacand).

- **Angiotensin receptor plus neprilysin inhibitors (ARNIs).** This medicine uses two blood pressure drugs to treat heart failure. The combination medicine is sacubitril-valsartan (Entresto). It's used to treat some people with heart failure with reduced ejection fraction. It may help prevent the need for a hospital stay in those people.

- **Beta blockers.** These medicines slow the heart rate and lower blood pressure. They reduce the symptoms of heart failure and help the heart work better.

If you have heart failure, beta blockers may help you live longer. Examples include carvedilol (Coreg), metoprolol (Lopressor, Toprol-XL, Kapspargo Sprinkle) and bisoprolol.

- **Diuretics.** Often called water pills, these medicines make you urinate more frequently. This helps prevent fluid buildup in your body. Diuretics, such as furosemide (Lasix, Furoscix), also decrease fluid in the lungs, so it's easier to breathe.

Some diuretics make the body lose potassium and magnesium. Your health care provider may recommend supplements to treat this. If you're taking a diuretic, you may have regular blood tests to check your potassium and magnesium levels.

- **Potassium-sparing diuretics.** Also called aldosterone antagonists, these drugs include spironolactone (Aldactone, Carospir) and eplerenone (Inspra). They may help people with severe heart failure with reduced ejection fraction (HFrEF) live longer.

Unlike some other diuretics, these medicines can raise the level of potassium in the blood to dangerous levels. Talk to your health care provider about your diet and potassium intake.

- **Sodium-glucose cotransporter-2 (SGLT2) inhibitors.** These medicines help lower blood sugar. They are often prescribed with diet and exercise to treat type 2 diabetes. But they're also one of the first treatments for heart failure. That's because several studies showed that the medicine lowered the risk of hospital stays and death in people with certain types of heart failure — even if they didn't have diabetes. These medicines include canagliflozin (Invokana), dapagliflozin (Farxiga), and empagliflozin (Jardiance).

- **Digoxin (Lanoxin).** This drug, also called digitalis, helps the heart squeeze better to pump blood. It also tends to slow the heartbeat. Digoxin reduces heart failure symptoms in people with HFrEF. It may be more likely to be given to someone with a heart

rhythm problem, such as atrial
fibrillation.

- **Hydralazine and isosorbide dinitrate (BiDil).** This drug combination helps relax blood vessels. It may be added to your treatment plan if you have severe heart failure symptoms and ACE inhibitors or beta blockers haven't helped.

- **Vericiguat (Verquvo).** This medicine for chronic heart failure is taken once a day by mouth. It's a type of drug called an oral soluble guanylate cyclase (sGC) stimulator. In studies, people with high-risk heart failure who took this medicine had fewer hospital stays for heart failure and heart disease-related deaths compared with those who got a dummy pill.

- **Positive inotropes.** These medicines may be given by IV to people with certain types of severe heart failure who are in the hospital. Positive inotropes can help the heart pump blood better and maintain blood pressure. Long-term use of these medicines has been linked to an increased risk of death in some people. Talk to your health care provider about the benefits and risks of these drugs.

- **Other medicines.** Your health care provider may prescribe other medicines to treat specific symptoms. For example, some people may receive nitrates for chest pain, statins to lower cholesterol or blood thinners to help prevent blood clots.

Arrhythmias

Atrial Fibrillation

Atrial fibrillation, often known as AFib, is an abnormal cardiac rhythm that is frequently very fast. An irregular heartbeat is medically referred to as having an arrhythmia. AFib has been linked to the formation of blood clots in the heart. The disorder also raises one's probability of suffering a stroke, heart failure, and several other issues connected to the heart.

Atrial fibrillation is characterized by erratic and disorganized beating of the upper chambers of the heart, which are known as the atria. They did not beat in time with the bottom chambers of the heart, which are known as ventricles. AFib may not present any symptoms at all in many patients. But atrial fibrillation can lead to symptoms such as a rapid and pounding heartbeat, difficulty breathing, or dizziness.

Atrial fibrillation may occur in episodes that come and go, or it may be a continuous condition. In most cases, having AFib does not pose a significant risk to one's life. However, being a significant medical disease, it requires treatment in order to reduce the risk of having a stroke.

Medications, therapies designed to shock the heart back into a normal rhythm, and surgical procedures designed to block erroneous cardiac impulses are all potential treatments for atrial fibrillation.

Atrial flutter is a similar cardiac rhythm disorder that may also be present in a person who has been diagnosed with atrial fibrillation. Both atrial fibrillation and atrial flutter are treated in a similar manner.

Symptoms

Symptoms of AFib may include:

- Feelings of a fast, fluttering or pounding heartbeat, called palpitations.

- Chest pain.

- Dizziness.

- Fatigue.

- Lightheadedness.

- Reduced ability to exercise.

- Shortness of breath.

- Weakness.

Some people with atrial fibrillation (AFib) don't notice any symptoms.

Atrial fibrillation may be:

- **Occasional, also called paroxysmal atrial fibrillation.** AFib symptoms come and go. The symptoms usually last for a few minutes to hours. Some people have symptoms for as long as a week. The episodes can happen repeatedly. Symptoms might go away on their own. Some people with occasional AFib need treatment.

- **Persistent.** The irregular heartbeat is constant. The heart rhythm does not reset on its own. If symptoms occur, medical treatment is needed to correct the heart rhythm.

- **Long-standing persistent.** This type of AFib is constant and lasts longer than 12 months. Medicines or a procedure are needed to correct the irregular heartbeat.

- **Permanent.** In this type of atrial fibrillation, the irregular heart rhythm can't be reset. Medicines are needed to control the heart rate and to prevent blood clots.

Causes

To understand the causes of atrial fibrillation (AFib), it may be helpful to know how the heart typically beats.

The heart has four chambers:

- The two upper chambers are called the atria.

- The two lower chambers are called the ventricles.

Inside the upper right heart chamber is a group of cells called the sinus node. The sinus node makes the signals that starts each heartbeat.

The signals move across the upper heart chambers. Next, the signals arrive at a group of cells called the AV node, where they usually slow down. The signals then go to the lower heart chambers.

In a healthy heart, this signaling process usually goes smoothly. The resting heart rate is typically 60 to 100 beats a minute.

But in atrial fibrillation, the signals in the upper chambers of the heart are chaotic. As a result, the upper chambers tremble or shake. The AV node is flooded with signals trying to get through to the lower heart chambers. This causes a fast and irregular heart rhythm.

In people with AFib, the heart rate may range from 100 to 175 beats a minute.

Causes of atrial fibrillation

Problems with the heart's structure are the most common cause of atrial fibrillation (AFib).

Heart diseases and health problems that can cause AFib include:

- A heart problem you're born with, called a congenital heart defect.

- A problem with the heart's natural pacemaker, called sick sinus syndrome.

- A sleep disorder called obstructive sleep apnea.

- Heart attack.

- Heart valve disease.

- High blood pressure.

- Lung diseases, including pneumonia.

- Narrowed or blocked arteries, called coronary artery disease.

- Thyroid disease such as an overactive thyroid.

- Infections from viruses.

Heart surgery or stress due to surgery or sickness may also cause AFib. Some people who have atrial fibrillation have no known heart disease or heart damage.

Lifestyle habits that can trigger an AFib episode may include:

- Drinking too much alcohol or caffeine.

- Illegal drug use.

- Smoking or using tobacco.

- Taking medicines that contain stimulants, including cold and allergy medicines bought without a prescription.

Prevention

Healthy lifestyle choices can reduce the risk of heart disease and may prevent atrial fibrillation (AFib).

Here are some basic heart-healthy tips:

Control high blood pressure, high cholesterol and diabetes.

Don't smoke or use tobacco.

Eat a diet that's low in salt and saturated fat.

Exercise at least 30 minutes a day on most days of the week unless your health care team says not to.

Get good sleep. Adults should aim for 7 to 9 hours daily.

Maintain a healthy weight.

Reduce and manage stress.

Structural Heart Conditions

Valvular Heart Disease

In the condition known as heart valve disease, one or more of the heart's valves do not function as they should. There are four valves located in the heart. They ensure that the blood continues to flow through the heart in the appropriate direction. There are occasions in which a valve does not open or close completely. Because of this, the way blood travels through the heart and out to the rest of the body may be altered.

Treatment for heart valve illness is contingent on the particular heart valve that is afflicted, as well as the nature and degree of the disease. When a heart valve needs to be repaired or replaced, surgery is sometimes required.

Symptoms

Some people with heart valve disease might not have symptoms for many years. When symptoms occur, they might include:

- Shortness of breath at rest or when active or lying down.

- Fatigue.

- Chest pain.

- Dizziness.

- Swelling of the ankles and feet.

- Fainting.

- Irregular heartbeat.

Causes

To understand the causes of heart valve disease, it may be helpful to know how the heart works.

Four valves in the heart keep blood flowing in the right direction. These valves are:

- Aortic valve.

- Mitral valve.

- Pulmonary valve.

- Tricuspid valve.

Each valve has flaps, called leaflets or cusps. The flaps open and close once during each heartbeat. If a valve flap doesn't open or close properly, less blood moves out of the heart to the rest of the body.

Types of heart valve disease include:

- **Stenosis.** The valve flaps become thick or stiff and sometimes can join together. The valve opening becomes narrowed. Less blood can flow through the narrowed valve.

- **Regurgitation.** The valve flaps may not close tightly, causing blood to leak backward.

- **Prolapse.** The valve flaps become stretched out and floppy. They bulge backward like a parachute. This condition can lead to regurgitation.

- **Atresia.** The valve isn't formed. A solid sheet of tissue blocks the blood flow between the heart chambers. This type usually affects the pulmonary valve.

Some people are born with heart valve disease. This is called congenital heart valve disease. But adults can get heart valve disease too. Causes of heart valve disease in adults may include infections, age-related changes and other heart conditions.

Diagnosis

To diagnose heart valve disease, a health care professional examines you and asks questions about your symptoms and health history. A whooshing sound called a heart murmur may be heard when listening to your heart with a device called a stethoscope.

Blood and imaging tests may be done to check your heart health.

Tests

Tests to diagnose heart valve disease may include:

- **Echocardiogram.** This test uses sound waves to create pictures of the beating heart. It shows how blood flows through the heart and the health of the heart valves. There are different types of echocardiograms. The type you have depends on the reason for the test and your overall health.

- **Electrocardiogram (ECG or EKG).** This quick test records the electrical signals in the heart. It shows how the heart is beating. Sensors, called electrodes, are attached to the chest and sometimes the legs. Wires connect the sensors to a computer, which displays or prints results.

- **Chest X-ray.** A chest X-ray shows the heart and lungs. The test can tell if the heart is larger than usual or if there is fluid around the lungs. Fluid could be due to some types of heart valve disease.

- **Cardiac MRI.** A cardiac MRI uses magnetic fields and radio waves to create detailed images of the heart. It can help determine the severity of heart valve disease.

- **Exercise tests or stress tests.** These tests often involve walking on a treadmill or riding a stationary bike while the heart is checked. Exercise tests show how the heart responds to physical activity and whether valve disease symptoms occur during exercise. If you can't exercise, you might get medicines that mimic the effect of exercise on the heart.

- **Cardiac catheterization.** This test isn't often used to diagnose heart valve disease. But it may be done if other tests can't diagnose a heart valve problem. Or it might be used to tell how severe heart valve disease is. A long, thin flexible tube called a catheter is inserted in a blood vessel, usually in the groin or wrist. It's guided to the heart. Dye flows through the catheter into the arteries in the heart. The dye helps the arteries show up more clearly on X-ray images and video.

Heart valve disease stages

After testing confirms a diagnosis of heart valve disease, your health care team may tell you the stage of disease. Staging helps determine the most appropriate treatment.

The stage of heart valve disease depends on many things, including symptoms, disease severity, the structure of the valve or valves, and blood flow through the heart and lungs.

Heart valve disease is staged into four basic groups:

- **Stage A: At risk.** Risk factors for heart valve disease are present.

- **Stage B: Progressive.** Valve disease is mild or moderate. There are no heart valve symptoms.

- **Stage C: Asymptomatic severe.** There are no heart valve symptoms but the valve disease is severe.

- **Stage D: Symptomatic severe.** Heart valve disease is severe and is causing symptoms.

Treatment

Heart valve disease treatment depends on:

- The symptoms.

- The severity of the disease.

- If the heart valve problem is getting worse.

Treatment may include:

- Regular health checkups.

- Lifestyle and diet changes.

- Medicines.

- Surgery to repair or replace the valve.

Medications

Some people with heart valve disease need medicines to treat their symptoms. Blood thinners may be given to help prevent blood clots.

Surgery or other procedures

A diseased or damaged heart valve might eventually need to be repaired or replaced, even if you don't have symptoms.

If you need surgery for another heart condition, a surgeon might do valve repair or replacement at the same time.

Methods to repair or replace heart valves include open-heart surgery or minimally invasive heart surgery. Surgeons at some medical centers may do robot-assisted heart valve surgery. The type of heart valve surgery done depends on many things, including age, overall health, and the type and severity of heart valve disease.

Heart valve repair

If you have heart valve disease, your health care team might suggest surgery to repair and save your heart valve. During heart valve repair, the surgeon might:

- Patch holes in a valve.

- Separate valve flaps that have connected.

- Repair the structure of the valve by replacing torn or ruptured cords that support it.

- Remove excess valve tissue so that the valve can close tightly.

- Reduce the outer size of the valve so the flaps can better contact each other.

Heart valve repair procedures include:

- **Annuloplasty.** A surgeon tightens or reinforces the outer ring around the valve. This surgery may be done with other treatments to repair a heart valve.

- **Valvuloplasty.** This surgery is used to repair the flaps of the valve. It's often done to repair mitral valve prolapse. The surgeon inserts a flexible tube with a balloon on the tip into an artery in the arm or groin area. The surgeon guides the tube to the affected heart valve. The balloon is inflated. This widens the valve opening. The balloon is deflated, and the tube and balloon are removed. Sometimes clips or plugs are passed through the tube to repair the heart valve.

Heart valve replacement

If a heart valve can't be repaired, surgery may be done to replace it. The most commonly replaced valves are the mitral and aortic valves. A surgeon removes the damaged heart valve and replaces it with one of the following:

- **A mechanical valve.** This type of artificial heart valve is made of strong material. It also is called a manufactured valve. If you have a mechanical valve, you need blood thinners for life to prevent blood clots.

- **A biological valve.** This type of artificial heart valve is made from cow, pig or human heart tissue. Biological tissue valves break down over time and eventually need to be replaced.

Sometimes, the aortic valve is replaced with the person's own pulmonary valve. Then the pulmonary valve is replaced with a biological valve. This more complicated surgery is called the Ross procedure.

Valve replacement typically requires open-heart surgery. But less invasive procedures may be available, depending on which heart valve is affected. For example, if the aortic valve is narrowed, surgeons may do transcatheter aortic valve replacement

(TAVR). It uses smaller incisions than those used in open-heart surgery.

Preventive Measures

Hypertension Control

If you have high blood pressure, you may be curious about whether or not taking medication to bring the numbers down is required. However, altering one's way of life is an essential component of hypertension management. By maintaining a healthy lifestyle, blood pressure can be managed, thereby eliminating, delaying, or reducing the need for medication.

1. Lose extra pounds and watch your waistline

When a person gains weight, their blood pressure will often rise. Being overweight also increases your risk of developing a condition known as sleep apnea, which disrupts your breathing while you are asleep and contributes further to high blood pressure.

Losing weight is one of the most effective adjustments in lifestyle that can be made to